The Healthy Belly Solution

Dale Downs

Dedication

Thanks to my family, friends, co-workers, teachers, professors, fellow basketball players, flight instructors, rodeo community, and pastors for being a part of the many diverse experiences I have had in my life. All of you are part of my foundation that motivated me to write this publication. Special thanks to Heidi for challenging my procrastination.

What is This All About?

The Healthy Belly Solution aims to empower you with knowledge and practical strategies for achieving and maintaining a lean and healthy lifestyle through self-managed dietary choices. Unlike many approaches that rely on branded foods, expensive supplements, strenuous exercise routines, or costly prescriptions, our focus is on simple, sustainable dietary management. In fact, with the right nutritional choices, you can achieve remarkable results with just 15 to 30 minutes of exercise four days a week. The key takeaway: achieving a healthy, lean body doesn't require extreme workouts or highly restrictive diet plans when you commit to sensible nutrition management.

Dispelling Diet Myths and Clarifying Information

In the following pages, we'll debunk common diet myths and cut through the noise of confusing information that bombards us daily. The internet can be a great tool for accessing good information quickly; it can also give us conflicting and even bad information at the same speed, especially regarding human nutrition. Drawing from extensive research, consultations, and presentations on nutrition, we'll provide you with valuable insights into the biological responses that occur when you consume different foods. Understanding these principles will empower you to make informed food choices, considering their impact on your body composition and overall health. We'll cover foundational knowledge and essential concepts regarding nutrition. However, the most critical path to success in achieving and maintaining a lean, youthful body is ensuring that your diet is manageable and aligns seamlessly with your daily life.

The Pitfall of Restrictive Diets

Nutrition and life congruence. Many "diets" and programs miss this critical factor, rendering them ineffective or suitable only for short-term results. While it's tempting to categorize foods as "must-eat" or "must-avoid," such an approach often leads to unmanageable situations. During a consult a few years back, the client stated, "I can't just go back and un-taste some of these foods. I love them." To present her comment another way, we can't erase our past food experiences or eliminate our cravings for certain indulgent treats. The reality is that we are continually exposed to foods we enjoy, even if they aren't technically part of a strict diet plan. The solution? Focus on consuming foods based on straightforward percentages from well-defined categories. A wise friend once noted that the desire for familiar and beloved foods can be challenging to overcome. The journey to sustainable health should not mean permanently giving up these foods—it's simply not manageable. This is precisely why we've created a system of food categories.

Our Approach

The Healthy Belly Solution will guide you in discovering which foods your body naturally favors and why. We've designed a straightforward system that simplifies food categorization, allowing you to enjoy a diverse and appealing range of foods.

A New Perspective on Food and Drink

Consider the foods and drinks at your disposal as percentages of your weekly dietary intake rather than rigid restrictions. This flexible approach lets you make choices that align with your preferences and lifestyle while working towards your health and fitness goals.

We will revisit this later, and I will explain this simple concept in more detail and discuss where common foods and drinks fit into these categories.

Why Listen to Me?

Hello there! My name is Dale Downs, and I call Omaha, Nebraska, my home. Before I dive into my story, I'd like to share a little history. It all started when I hit the big 3-0, and I made a decision that might sound a bit unusual: I decided to transition my lifestyle. What triggered this change? Well, it was the simple act of shaving that got me thinking. Shaving forces you to stand shirtless in front of a mirror to avoid making a mess with water and shaving cream. During one of these morning rituals, while I was frequently on the road due to my heavy travel schedule, I couldn't help but wonder where my once-lean physique had disappeared to. That's when I began noticing my eating habits more. I looked in the mirror and did not like what I saw.

Making the Connection

Speaking of travel, let me share a little tip: avoid buying convenience foods on the go. Recently, a friend of mine embarked on an 8-hour journey and opted to pack healthy snacks at home instead of settling for less nutritious options along the way. Then, he could sit down for a nice meal when he arrived at his destination. This is a very basic but impactful change in habit for those who travel.

My College Days

Rewind seven years before that jarring encounter with my reflection, and you'd find me as an active undergraduate with single-digit body fat percentages. I once believed that age might be a valid excuse for changes in my physique, but now that I am in my early 50's, I've come to realize two things: 1) 50 is not old, and 2) age should never be an excuse. Can anyone else relate to wondering where that youthful, lean body went?

A Promise to You

I'm thrilled you've chosen to read this because it doesn't have to be this way, and I want to emphasize that age should never hold you back. You don't have to accept the "American Pot Belly" as the norm.

My Turning Point

To provide some context, early in our marriage, my then-wife and I had fallen into a sedentary lifestyle, and our dietary choices were nothing short of terrible. That's when I decided to take matters into my own hands. Armed with knowledge of physiology, the endocrine system, and more, I shed nearly 30 pounds of excess fat. However, this transformation raised eyebrows among friends and family, who thought I needed medical attention. My doctor's response was eye-opening: "You're in excellent condition; the problem is that Americans aren't accustomed to seeing people with proper amounts of body fat." A sobering truth, indeed.

Reaping the Rewards

As the excess weight melted away, I felt the magic happening. My joints felt better, my energy levels soared, and I rediscovered the joy of activities like running, jumping, and playing basketball 3 to 4 times a week, alongside strength training. Once I experienced how good I could feel, I vowed never to return to my previous state. This commitment fueled my passion for understanding human nutrition and fitness. Even my wife (now my ex), Kathe, joined in with an impressive 80-pound weight loss. **At ages 52 and 50, we proudly maintain the lean builds we had back in our college days.**

My Background in Nutrition

Growing up on a farm and ranch in Western Nebraska, earning an MS in animal nutrition, and spending the first 15 years of my career focused on making animals grow efficiently gave me unique insights. It became clear why people's habits and food choices were contributing to America's obesity and health problems. It is much more difficult to conduct research and understand cause-and-effect relationships in humans due to free will and diversity in lifestyle. In other words, when we study the response to dietary variables in animals, we control what they eat and their environment as much as possible. This is very difficult, if not impossible, with humans, so human nutrition science could be termed as less pure than animal science. I was therefore inspired to seek clarity in human nutrition using my background with animals, free from the propaganda in the human diet industry. I then used myself as the guinea pig.

A Battle Against Hypocrisy

I faced a personal struggle with hypocrisy. How could I, armed with knowledge about why animals gain fat, continue with poor habits? Additionally, I was consulting on nutrition, albeit for animals. I realized that I couldn't effectively help others manage their livelihoods in animal production if I wasn't managing my own health and fitness.

A Passion for Nutrition and Exercise

So, I embarked on a journey to integrate dietary fundamentals into our household. I taught myself to cook healthily, and Kathe and I both developed a passion for nutrition and exercise. In the meantime, she achieved her black belt in karate, became a NASM-certified trainer, and opened two fitness facilities.

The Quest for Truth

Since I started my transformation, I've devoted significant time to understanding the truth about human habits and nutrition. What I discovered often contradicted the advice given by the government, so-called experts, and the food and diet industry over several decades. It's not always intuitive, but in this short read, I'll share what I've learned.

The Possibility of Dietary Management

Dietary management is possible, even for someone like me, who sometimes has a short attention span and a busy life running companies. I'm also the proud father of two boys, Max and Luke, and I am remarried to an amazing lady, Heidi.

Dispelling Diet Myths and Clarifying Information

What Should I Eat?

Now, this is a question I've been asked countless times by friends and colleagues who've noticed my dedication to solid nutritional principles. I believe the so-called "magic" dietary supplement lies in education and a touch of discipline. It's high time we dispel the myths and unravel the confusion created by the food, diet, and medical industry. Let's put an end to the misery, expense, and inefficacy of dietary management.

The Truth Shall Set You Free

I firmly believe that truth and knowledge can empower you to take control of your life, particularly when managing your diet. You don't need to follow a pre-packaged diet plan or obsessively hit the gym to achieve your health goals. I greatly respect fitness enthusiasts, trainers, and dietitians, but not everyone can—or should—dedicate their entire lives to these pursuits.

Balancing Act

Often, advice from those deeply immersed in nutrition and fitness can be overwhelming for individuals who approach these aspects of life on a "part-time" basis. That's why I've tagged this publication as the "Path to Nutritional Autonomy." Autonomy means independence or freedom in decision-making, and this is all about achieving Nutritional Sovereignty. For the purists out there, rest assured that I won't delve into scientific jargon or cite endless studies. I aim to provide you with practical and applicable insights, not to publish a scholarly article.

Disclaimer

Before we continue, a quick disclaimer: if bacon happens to be linked to any unfortunate events, it's not my doing. Additionally, you may encounter opinions and observations within this book that you respectfully disagree with. That's perfectly okay. The views discussed, however, have proven to be effective.

Why Manage Our Diet?

Back in the day, our dietary choices were dictated by what could be hunted, grown, or gathered in another way from nature. Times have changed. Modern society has made an abundance of highly concentrated foods rich in poor nutrients readily available—sometimes to our detriment. Take sugar, for instance. It was virtually impossible in the past to consume the equivalent of 234 grams of pure sugar in a 64-ounce cola in a reasonable amount of time. Today, we can down that soda in minutes, despite it taking nearly 52 pounds of sugar cane to produce that much pure sugar. To confess, when I was traveling for my first occupation, I would commonly consume two 32-ounce sodas fully loaded with sugar, which is why I wanted to understand this calculation. Our bodies weren't designed for these dietary choices, and it's reflected in our body fat percentages.

The Benefits of a Healthy Body

Maintaining a healthy body fat percentage offers numerous advantages. It enhances self-image, reduces stress on joints, decreases the risk of medical issues, and boosts energy levels, just to name a few.

Changing Times

In the past, lifestyle and food availability were primarily shaped by the environment rather than humans dictating the environment. This paradigm has shifted, posing a new challenge.

The Junk Food Epidemic

The majority of what we now consider "staples" in grocery stores and restaurants can be classified as junk food. The low production cost and substantial profit margins associated with items like flour and soybean oil have led to an influx of heavily processed, convenient foods. These products often contain ingredients and chemically manufactured substances that our bodies struggle to process and don't even recognize as nutrients.

A Look into Fast Food

Let's talk about fast food, shall we? While I'm not here to single out any specific fast-food chain, I can't help but wonder how it's possible that the price of a hamburger has increased by less than 80% over 30 years, despite ground beef costs rising nearly 100% minimum wage more than doubling, and travel expenses (as indicated by IRS mileage reimbursement rates) more than doubling as well. The Consumer Price Index has also increased over two-fold during this period. The math doesn't quite add up.

Unraveling Fast Food

Even if my calculations aren't exact, the fact remains: fast food often includes excessive bread and minimal meat, served alongside side items built from inexpensive, unhealthy ingredients. These side items include French fries fried in unhealthy vegetable oils, sugary sodas, and shakes that contain more sugar than cream. Some chains even have level pricing between a small soda and a large, which influences people to consume more because of the perceived value. Most chain delis follow a similar pattern.

The Taste Extremes

I have no qualms about enjoying a burger, but it seems that many fast-food burgers have become a bun with a smattering of meat rather than the other way around. The disparities in pricing within the fast-food industry over the years, as well as the ingredients used to create taste extremes and consequential cravings, raise questions. One example is the extensive use of Monosodium Glutamate, a flavor enhancer that has been linked to obesity. I do not think the compound itself influences body fat. However, I believe the craving increases for foods that contain significant levels.

4

An Unhealthy Culprit

Most people are aware that downing a supersized soda and fries isn't a wise choice. However, by the end of this book, I hope to shed light on just how detrimental some of these ingredients can be for your body. Beyond contributing to fat accumulation, certain ingredients found in fast food can cause inflammation and wreak havoc on your health.

A Dietary Dilemma

The United States, as great as it is, faces a dietary crisis. Our dietary flame has been fueled in part by the flawed philosophy behind the old FDA food pyramid—the one with bread, cereal, rice, and pasta forming the foundation while fats and oils barely cling to the top. Many of us were taught this pyramid in elementary school.

Fueling the Fire

Readily available, inexpensive "foods" dense in the wrong nutrients only add fuel to the dietary fire. Bad advice from the medical community, our susceptibility to certain tastes, and misleading marketing tactics employed by food companies have turned this situation into an inferno. Some of the health claims found on food packaging, especially for unhealthy items, are nothing short of scandalous. If these claims were on animal feed labels, they'd likely be heavily scrutinized.

Taking Charge

Given all these factors, the saying "if it's to be, it's up to me" applies here. To limit our propensity for obesity, chronic pain, and disease, we must make dietary management an integral part of our daily lives. Nobody else will do it for us, and the cultural norms are stacked against us.

Wrap Your Mind Around It!

Contrary to popular belief, the manifestation of excess body fat is not solely determined by genetics. To unravel the intricate web of factors influencing lean-to-fat ratios, we must examine the roles played by food, activity, and genetics. Astonishingly, food contributes around 70-75%, activity around 20-25%, and genetics around 5-10%. While genetic predispositions may exist, environmental factors and dietary choices significantly influence their actual impact, especially regarding fat deposition.

Venturing into the fascinating domain of nutri-genomics, an evolving science exploring the interplay between food nutrients and gene expression, sheds light on the profound impact of food choices on gene expression. Despite being in its early stages, nutrigenomics challenges the misconception that genetics rigidly dictates fate. It's time to recognize that you have the power to shape your health through conscious dietary decisions.

Dispelling the myth, it's crucial to acknowledge that not all fats contribute to weight gain. Proper fats are essential nutrients, and envisioning a scenario on a desert island underscores the importance of fats alongside water for survival. Unlike simple carbohydrates that trigger insulin spikes and hinder fat loss, fat consumption is an essential part of a healthy diet.

When considering the totality of macro and micronutrients in foods, the sum must always equal 100%. Reducing fat content often leads to an influx of sugars and simple carbohydrates, emphasizing the need for a transition to a fat-burning metabolism, particularly for those accustomed to diets that are high in starch and sugar—a prevalent trend in American eating habits.

The long-standing vilification of dietary cholesterol and saturated fats is gradually losing ground. This notion limited consumption of many amazing foods for years. The connection between dietary cholesterol, saturated fats, and heart disease was built on biased and flawed science. Undoing such deeply rooted beliefs takes time, but a paradigm shift is underway.

Circulating cholesterol levels alone provide an incomplete picture. Considering inflammation induced by inflammatory foods and environmental factors is equally crucial. LDL cholesterol, frequently demonized, is comprised of various particle sizes and densities with different behaviors in the body. Some saturated fats do not negatively influence cholesterol profile, and understanding the distinction between cholesterol particle sizes is essential for a comprehensive assessment.

The next time your physician recommends a cholesterol test, insist on a particle test for a more accurate evaluation. A particle test differentiates particle size within HDL and LDL for interpretation of potential consequences within the body. Cholesterol is highly regulated within the body through a complex process, and natural production is changed based on cholesterol consumption. Before opting for statin medications, it's important to weigh their implications—these drugs are not a universal solution, and the risks of overprescription must be considered. Cholesterol doing its job is not the problem in the cardiovascular system. Rather, it is bodily assault from ingestion of inflammatory foods and toxins.

I have consulted with many who were on or destined for cholesterol and blood pressure medications who avoided them entirely through dietary management. Type 2 diabetes can also generally be controlled through diet.

The cholesterol and saturated fat paradigm has had far-reaching consequences, leading to the avoidance of nutritious foods such as meat, egg yolks, and saturated fats such as butter, while causing a sharp rise in manufactured health-damaging alternatives. Questioning food labels boasting health claims, and delving into the actual ingredients and nutritional profiles empower you to navigate through the noise and make decisions that genuinely benefit your body. Armed with knowledge, you become the architect of your health journey.

Calories & Nutrient Density

Your mother's wisdom rings true: "Do not eat empty calories." However, my focus extends beyond mere calorie counting; it emphasizes selecting nutrient-dense foods that align with your body's needs. Nutrient density refers to foods where the majority of nutrients are meaningful and synergize with your body—a classification I dub "Good" in my food categorization.

Empty foods, on the other hand, negatively impact blood sugar management without offering substantial nutrients that enhance biological function and body composition. Even within a reasonable calorie intake, consuming inflammatory, adulterated foods can impede weight and body composition goals. These foods trigger inflammation and hormonal responses that transcend the simplistic calories in/calories out philosophy. Healthy fats, which are essential, contain roughly double the calories of simple carbohydrates, which are not essential. Calories in/calories out has been proven to be ineffective as a long-term dietary management strategy in most cases. If dietary management were only about calories, we could consume 10 to 15 twelve-ounce sodas and be perfectly healthy.

The crucial takeaway is that not all calories are created equal. While this doesn't endorse food excess, adhering to the principles outlined in this book makes responsible food intake more manageable. Personally, I only scrutinize calorie content when simple carbohydrates dominate the composition.

Hormones & Biochemistry

The primary aim of "The Healthy Belly Solution" is to equip you with information for personalized nutrition management. To achieve this, you need a reference point and a basic understanding of fundamental food choices, coupled with insights into the consequences of poor dietary decisions on your body's biochemistry.

Although hormones and biochemistry involve complex processes beyond exhaustive discussion here, I'll highlight key concepts we'll reference in discussions about specific foods later. As you implement the teachings from "The Healthy Belly Solution," you'll alter the dynamics of your endocrine (hormonal) system through dietary choices.

Understanding the basics of hormones and body fat storage/loss reinforces effective management. Terms like glycemic index, glycemic load, insulin, and insulin resistance are likely familiar, and they all tie into the management of blood sugar, circulating insulin, and the crucial prevention of consistent insulin spikes.

Managing blood sugar is pivotal for fat-burning and maintaining leanness. When you consume a simple carbohydrate-heavy meal, insulin rushes in to move sugar from the bloodstream into muscle cells. If these cells don't need the energy, insulin and its assistant LPL (lipoprotein lipase) shuttle the sugar into fat cells. This highlights that it is sugar, not dietary fat, that contributes to fat accumulation.

Fat burning becomes difficult in a high blood sugar state, with insulin doing its job. Another hormone, glucagon, which signals the release of stored fat for energy, is suppressed. In the presence of high blood sugar and insulin, glucagon and its helper HSL (hormone-sensitive lipase) can't efficiently break down stored fat into usable energy.

Constant spikes in blood sugar and subsequent insulin levels not only lead to unwanted body fat but also contribute to inflammatory diseases like cardiovascular disease and cancer. Sugars, particularly refined sugars, play a role in free radical damage and degenerative aging. All non-fiber carbohydrates convert to sugar in the bloodstream. The overconsumption of refined sugars may prove to be more impactful on inflammatory diseases than tobacco in the future.

While life offers no guarantees, understanding and exerting control over dietary choices can significantly influence health outcomes.

Nerves and Microbes

Why does our entire body feel bad when our gut is out of whack? An often-overlooked fact is that the enteric nervous system, a massive network of neurons in our digestive system, has a profound interaction with the brain. The enteric nervous system contains more neurons than exist in either the peripheral nervous system or the spinal cord. This system can control gut behavior independent of the brain and has two-way communication. For example, sometimes, when we are nervous, we may experience butterflies in our stomach (a signal to the brain). If we are feeling depressed or stressed, we may have an upset stomach (signal from the brain). An upset stomach or constipation due to poor dietary management can cause many negative symptoms throughout the body, including changes in mood. A signal from the gut tells the brain when we are experiencing G-Force.

Microbes in the digestive system of humans and animals are also an extremely important consideration when it comes to health and performance. The gut microflora is comprised of mostly bacteria, both good and bad. One can help boost gut health though supplementation of prebiotics and/or probiotics. Prebiotics help naturally occurring good bacteria gain an advantage over bad bacteria. Probiotics are direct supplementation of beneficial bacteria. Many fermented foods and drinks result in natural probiotic bacterial cultures. One example is apple cider vinegar with "The Mother." A shot of this every day is a little rough on the taste buds, but something your body loves. Kombucha, a fermented tea, may be a little more tolerable to get a nice dose of probiotic bacteria. Consuming foods and using the fundamentals outlined in this manuscript generally will result in a healthy microflora.

What's the point? Eating properly the majority of the time has a profound impact on our bodies beyond being lean.

Become a Fat Burner

In the realm of typical Western diets, overconsumption of non-fiber carbohydrates is pervasive. Simple carbohydrates like sugar, high fructose corn syrup, and refined flour swiftly elevate blood sugar levels. Others, with some fiber content, such as certain whole grains and beans, have a slower digestion rate and milder blood sugar response. Regardless, all simple carbohydrates eventually convert to sugar in the bloodstream.

The term "sugar burner" characterizes the metabolic state induced by diets heavily reliant on the aforementioned foods. In this state, the body heavily depends on blood sugar as its primary fuel source. Individuals programmed as sugar burners need frequent meals to sustain blood sugar levels, and their bodies predominantly rely on sugar for energy. The consequences of a drop in blood sugar include a rapid decline in both physical and mental performance, often leading to "Hangry" episodes.

Contrastingly, a body programmed as a "fat burner" relies on alternative fuel sources—ketones and free fatty acids derived from fats. Diets promoting fat burning entail sufficient consumption of healthy fats while minimizing sugar and starch-laden foods. Unlike sugar burners, individuals on a fat-burning diet experience sustained energy after meals, with insulin levels remaining stable. This stability allows the endocrine system to prepare the body to utilize stored fat for energy. Such dietary choices promote stable thinking and moods, slower aging, and reduced cravings. The prevalence of sugar burner metabolic programming is partly attributed to the low-fat dietary trend of recent decades.

Quit Wheat & Check Dairy

Wheat, a staple in many diets, warrants a closer look due to potential intolerances. Temporarily abstaining from wheat products for two weeks can reveal its impact on your well-being. Beyond gluten intolerance, wheat has been implicated in various issues, including addictive properties, increased food consumption, acne, joint degeneration, and potential links to irritable bowel syndrome and acid reflux. Moreover, wheat can spike blood sugar and contribute to the deposition of visceral fat, even in individuals without apparent intolerance. Regardless of tolerance levels, keeping wheat at a minimum in your diet is advisable.

Similarly, evaluating dairy consumption involves a temporary cessation to observe how it influences your body, independent of wheat. Opting for higher-fat dairy products is recommended, as low-fat alternatives often contain more sugar or artificial sweeteners and lack nutrient density. Scientifically, dairy fat has been shown to support fat loss efforts, contrary to popular belief. Fermented dairy products without added sugar can be a beneficial choice, offering valuable bacterial cultures.

Let's Talk Food & Drink

Categorizing available food and drink options based on loose percentages of your total diet over time provides a practical approach. Foods can fall into three categories: "Good," "Moderate," and "Limited."

"Good" foods, representing 75% or more of your diet, include those found along the exterior aisles of grocery stores, close to the farm, and with small ingredient lists.

"Moderate" foods make up about 15% of your diet, consumed 2-3 times per week.

"Limited" foods, constituting 5% or less of your diet, are treats and should be chosen sparingly, around one time per week.

"Avoid" foods are self-explanatory and should only be consumed when no other option exists.

These categories apply to various types of foods, such as drinks, meats, fats, vegetables, fruits, dairy items, side dishes, snacks, desserts, condiments, and grains. Prioritize choices aligning with the "Good" category for optimal health.

Drinks

Exercise caution when consuming liquid calories, as it's effortless to ingest hundreds or even thousands of empty calories in beverages. Water reigns supreme as the top choice, playing a foundational role in dietary management. Staying adequately hydrated is crucial for effective fat loss and maintaining leanness. Aim to consume between 0.66 and 1.0 ounces of water per pound of body weight per day, adjusting for activity levels and temperature. Typically, 3 to 6 liters per day should meet most individuals' water needs. Enhance the appeal of water by infusing it with lemons, limes, or other natural, low-calorie options. Creative solutions, such as pitchers with infusing compartments for cucumbers or fruit, add variety to plain water.

Once your hydration needs are met, consider incorporating teas and coffee into your routine. Adding a splash of heavy cream, half & half, or almond milk, sweetened with stevia if desired, can enhance these beverages. Both coffee and tea offer antioxidant benefits and have demonstrated positive effects on health. Opt for less processed caffeinated teas and coffee, avoiding heavily sweetened store-bought cappuccinos or lattes, which dilute the health benefits of coffee. A moderate amount of caffeine, particularly before a workout, can boost performance. Stevia complements acidic juices like lemon or lime, allowing you to create your own low-calorie lemonade or limeade. For those seeking variety, some flavored bottled drinks based on stevia can provide a refreshing alternative. If opting for a caloric drink, unsweetened almond and coconut milk are recommended, serving as excellent bases for nutrient-dense smoothies.

Meats, Other Protein Sources, Fats, & Oils

Meats: While lean meats are often recommended, a well-rounded diet includes both lean meats and those with fat, as meat serves as an excellent source of healthy fats. Fats from meats such as steak, brisket, ground beef, roast, chicken, turkey, bacon, pork belly, and quality bratwurst or sausage contribute to a balanced diet. For higher fat cuts of beef, grass-fed is a good choice, as there are differences in the fatty acid profile of the meat beneficial to the human body. Rub leaner meats with olive oil to retain moisture during cooking.

Eggs: Embrace eggs as a superfood and consume the entire egg, as the yolk contains valuable vitamins, minerals, good fats, and protein. Opt for farm-raised eggs with deep yellow yolks and opaque whites. Eggs can be prepared in various ways, adding versatility to your meals.

Protein Powders and Bars: Dairy-based proteins like whey isolate, whey concentrate, and milk protein concentrate, along with egg protein, are excellent choices. Plant-based sources such as peas, hemp seeds, chia seeds, and sprouted brown rice protein are suitable alternatives, while soy protein is excluded. When selecting protein powders or bars, prioritize those with minimal ingredients, natural non-sugar sweetening, and flavor. Remember that while these supplements can be convenient, the majority of nutrients should come from whole foods.

More on Dairy

For those with a good tolerance to dairy, fermented dairy products stand out as an excellent source of probiotics and protein. However, a careful examination of labels is essential. Fermented items like kefir and plain yogurts, with their naturally sour taste, can be targeted by manufacturers to sneak in excessive sugar or artificial sweeteners to cater to the Western palate's sweetness sensitivity. Exercise caution, especially with low and non-fat products. High-quality cheeses, such as Blue and Gorgonzola, are valuable additions to your diet, offering rich flavors and beneficial fats that provide satiety. Full-fat cottage cheese serves as a slow-release protein source, ideal for a bedtime snack or enhancing post-workout smoothies for added thickness, fat, and protein. Heavy cream and half & half can subtly enrich beverages. Opt for whole, unpasteurized, and non-homogenized milk when available. Alternatively, filtered milks are also viable options as they contain less milk sugar (lactose) and increased protein. Recommended brands will be shared in a forthcoming report.

Butter, a dairy product, is a commendable addition to your culinary arsenal. Avoid using butter replacements, as they contain inflammatory oils. Remember, dairy fat has been shown through scientific research, to assist in body fat loss.

Peanuts, Tree Nuts, and Seeds

This diverse group of foods, often unfairly scrutinized for their fat content and caloric density, offers superior nutritional density, delivering healthy fats, protein, fiber, and micronutrients. Without allergy concerns, these foods make excellent snacks and meal substitutes and serve as the basis for derivative products like oils, flours, butter, protein concentrates, and liquid milk. Ground nuts can create a wholesome crust for meat or fish or add a crunchy texture to salads or stir-fries.

Top choices within this category include pistachios, walnuts, almonds, macadamias, flax seeds, hemp seeds, chia seeds, sunflower seeds, and sesame seeds. Pecans, cashews, pine nuts, and peanuts are also viable options if allergies are not a concern. While both roasted and raw varieties are acceptable, raw nuts are preferable. Pay close attention to ingredient lists in roasted nuts, as potential additives will be addressed in the next sections.

Regarding nut oils, opt for minimally processed cold-pressed oils and butter. Choose oils based on flavor contribution and heat tolerance, with grapeseed, sesame, and nut oils suitable for high-heat cooking. Unrefined sunflower oil and other low-smoke point seed oils are better for uncooked applications. Purchase nut butter in its least processed form, and if possible, seek freshly made options available in many stores. Watch out for additives such as inflammatory oils and sugar in commercial nut butter, making label scrutiny crucial.

As a general rule, study the label to make informed choices. On a delightful note, the "Cracked Nut Butter" stands out as a superb product with a delightful taste, combining almond and pecan butter with whey protein isolate, stevia, and natural flavors. This low-sugar treat serves as an excellent dessert option. While there are various alternatives, "Cracked Nut Butter" is the best in terms of taste and nutritional profile, in my experience.

Avocados

These vibrant green gems truly earn their status as a superfood. It's surprising that some still limit their avocado intake due to concerns about the high-fat content. However, the monounsaturated fats in avocados are anti-inflammatory warriors, combating free radicals. These fats are susceptible to oxidation, causing avocados to turn brown when exposed to air. To preserve leftover avocados, leave the pit in, cover with citrus juice, wrap tightly, and refrigerate. For the guacamole, slice the avocado, remove the seed, smash the flesh, and add salsa, salt, pepper, and a hint of lime. Avocados are versatile and should be enjoyed daily, sliced with eggs, in smoothies, salads, or as a flavorful dressing for grilled meats. Avocado oil, with one of the highest smoke points among healthy oils, is also a fantastic source of fat.

Coconut

This divine drupe, loaded with healthy saturated fats (90%), offers extensive antioxidant properties, fighting cellular damage. It boasts health benefits like increased metabolism, anti-bacterial and anti-viral properties, skin aging reduction, improved digestion, blood sugar stabilization, hormonal regulation, weight loss assistance, and enhanced mental function. Coconut components include oil, flesh, water, and cream. Coconut oil is one of the healthiest cooking oils, ideal for stir-frying vegetables. Including a tablespoon or more in your daily diet is beneficial, especially for active individuals and athletes. Coconut cream is useful in cooking, popular in Thai curries, and can be part of a healthier ice cream treat. Shredded coconut meat serves as a versatile ingredient, from a breading alternative for chicken to ground flour for baking. Embrace all aspects of the coconut for a well-rounded inclusion in your diet.

Olives

A simple directive—enjoy all available varieties freely. Olive oil is excellent for dressings and cooking, handling heat well. Be discerning about the brand, as some olive oil producers may blend it with cheaper vegetable oils to cut costs.

Vegetables

This robust group of foods should grace every meal plate. It's important to note that while corn is often mistaken for a vegetable, it's actually a grain high in starch. Despite this, it can still find a place in the dietary plan but should be consumed in moderation. Opt for nutrient-rich choices like broccoli, cauliflower, green beans, asparagus, lettuce, celery, peas, and Brussels sprouts. Additionally, root vegetables such as potatoes, sweet potatoes, beets, carrots, onions, shallots, radishes, and garlic are all nutritious, but it's advisable to moderate the intake of starchy varieties like potatoes. Various preparation tips for these vegetables will be shared in my upcoming publication of "No-Measure Recipes."

Fruits

This diverse and delightful food group can be classified in two ways: botanically and culinarily. Here, I'll focus on the botanical classification, rooted in scientific principles. Some vegetables, from a botanical perspective, are also considered fruits, including avocados and olives (which have their own section), peas, and tomatoes. Tomatoes, in particular, provide numerous beneficial nutrients, including high levels of lycopene, a potent antioxidant known to prevent inflammatory diseases. Peppers of all kinds are also botanical fruits and offer various health benefits.

Another fruit classification includes pome fruits, with common examples being apples and pears—ideal choices for those seeking a slightly sweet and healthy option.

Tropical fruits encompass a wide range, including grapes, kiwi, guava, mango, cantaloupe, oranges, tangerines, lemons, limes, pomegranate, grapefruit, raspberries, blueberries, watermelon, and bananas. While watermelon has a higher sugar content, it boasts a low glycemic load, meaning it doesn't cause significant spikes in blood sugar despite its sweetness. These fruits, whether tropical or otherwise, offer natural sugars, hydration, and essential nutrients. Consider consuming higher-sugar fruits like bananas when your muscles need replenishing after intense physical activity. Limit consumption of fruit juices as fructose is concentrated in most commercial juices through processing.

In essence, all these fruits can be valuable components of a healthy and balanced diet.

Alcohol: A Balanced Approach

Approaching alcohol consumption with balance and mindfulness can contribute to a healthier lifestyle. When choosing to indulge in alcoholic beverages, moderation is key, and incorporating them into your evening meal can enhance the overall experience. Dry red wine stands out as a favorable choice, not only for its taste but also for the potential health benefits attributed to resveratrol, a potent antioxidant. For those seeking alternatives, clear liquors such as vodka and unsweetened whiskeys like Canadian,

Bourbon, Scotch, and Irish Whiskey provide sound options.

Steer clear of sweet liqueurs, as their high sugar content may contribute to fat deposition. As far as liquors, most of the weight gain demons live in the mixers. Opt for water, club soda, or unsweetened lemon/lime juice with a touch of stevia for sweetness. The combination of alcohol type and mixers can significantly influence fat retention, making it crucial to be mindful of choices, particularly when it comes to beer and simple carbs. Craft beers, rich in nutrients, offer a preferable option over lighter varieties, all while being mindful of caloric intake. A few good craft beers can be more satisfying and healthier than many light beers.

Sweeteners: Embrace the Natural

When it comes to sweeteners, a preference for unrefined options is a healthier choice. Even for those with a sweet tooth, the emphasis should be on choosing options close to nature. Consider incorporating sweeteners judiciously, especially in Asian cuisine and meat dishes, opting for pure maple syrup for its natural goodness. Raw honey, with its nutrient-rich profile, is a healthy choice, and locally-produced varieties may even assist in alleviating allergies. Stevia, a plant-derived non-caloric sweetener, serves as an excellent alternative to refined sugar and can be used in various culinary applications. While Agave Nectar is acceptable, it's essential to be aware that it may impact blood sugar more than other natural sweeteners. Almost anything can be made and taste great using the listed natural sweeteners.

Supplements: The Essentials

Think of essential supplements as your "fountain of youth," providing vital support for overall well-being:

- Selenium Yeast: This potent antioxidant has shown promise in regressing tumors in animals and works synergistically with Vitamin E to protect cells from oxidative damage.

- Turmeric/Curcumin: Beyond being an antioxidant, turmeric is a natural remedy for pain, widely used in Far East cuisines, contributing to the overall health of populations.

- Omega-3 Fatty Acids: Maintain a balance between omega-3 and omega-6 levels with fish oil or omega-3 supplements, supporting heart health and cognitive function.

- Vitamin D: This is especially crucial in regions with limited sun exposure; consider supplements to address deficiencies and promote bone health.

- B Complex: Essential for those with diets lacking in B12, especially for non-red meat consumers. Excess Water-soluble B Vitamins are generally excreted, so amounts need to be adequate but not exact.

- CoQ10: Assists in heart health, blood pressure regulation, and prevention of oxidative damage.

- Salt: Despite its association with health issues, salt is essential. Opt for Himalayan Pink Sea Salt, offering additional elements beyond sodium chloride, and use it judiciously in your cooking. Diets high in salt should also be higher in water consumption.

Remember, individual needs may vary, and it is advisable to consult with a healthcare professional before initiating any supplement regimen. Taking a holistic approach to your choices can pave the way for a well-balanced and health-conscious lifestyle.

Desserts: A Thoughtful Indulgence

Acknowledging that many desserts often contain ingredients that may not align with health goals, it's still possible to enjoy these treats occasionally while maintaining a commitment to staying lean. Opting for the previously recommended natural sweeteners and choosing butter over vegetable oil when feasible can make a significant difference. Select desserts that not only satisfy your sweet tooth but also provide essential nutrients, such as cheesecake, Crème Brûlée, and homemade ice cream. Be discerning in your choices, limiting options like donuts or pastries and favoring desserts that contribute positively to your overall well-being. While pies and cobblers, with their high refined sugar and flour content, should only be enjoyed in moderation, they can still be part of a balanced indulgence.

Reflecting on the tradition of dessert in a farm upbringing, where physical labor may have balanced the occasional treat, one realizes the importance of moderation and thoughtful ingredient choices.

Oils and Soybeans: Making Informed Choices

In the realm of cooking oils, awareness is paramount to making informed choices. Refined vegetable oils like canola, sunflower, and soybean, often present in processed foods, undergo extensive processing and may pose health risks, especially when used for high-temperature frying due to the release of free radicals. Soybean oil, since it is less expensive than most oils, is prevalent in many blends and processed foods. While suitable for non-human purposes like animal feed and biofuel, it should be kept at a minimum in human diets. It is the most common vegetable oil and the least healthy. The use of soybean-based foods in human nutrition is not advisable unless in roasted or fermented forms, such as in soy sauce. These oils, alongside soy products, may not align with the goals of those striving for a lean physique.

Refined Sugar: Know Your Limits

The pervasive consumption of refined sugar in Western culture contributes to various health concerns. While not entirely forbidden for those aiming to stay lean, its intake should be kept to a minimum. Scrutinize labels, be conscious of potential impacts on blood sugar levels, and choose wisely, understanding the consequences of the occasional indulgence.

High Fructose Corn Syrup: A Sweet Culprit

High fructose corn syrup, prevalent in processed foods and sodas, emerges as a significant contributor to elevated blood sugar levels. Limiting its consumption is crucial, given its potential adverse effects on hormones, as discussed earlier. Being aware of its impact is vital for individuals prioritizing their health.

Hydrogenated Oils: An Inflammatory Villain

Taking concerns about refined oils to a more concerning level, hydrogenated oils, resulting from the hydrogenation of vegetable oils, are frequently used for their shelf-life-extending properties. Found in numerous processed foods and many peanut butter brands, these oils contribute to inflammation and negatively impact overall health. Opting for nut butter with stable oils or palm oil and avoiding hydrogenated oils becomes crucial in steering clear of this inflammatory class of oils. Making informed choices about oils contributes to a healthier overall diet and supports the goals of individuals seeking to maintain a lean physique.

A Few Insights on General Nutrition

When and How Often Should We Eat:

This is a subject around which there are many mixed messages, so let's revisit your mother's nutritional advice to find clarity. As stated earlier, she was correct in her view to avoid eating empty calories. However, regarding breakfast being the most important meal of the day, which many mothers have stated, I respectfully disagree. Moms are seldom wrong, but my answer to the question on when to eat is that it does not matter in most cases. What matters is what is put in your body over the course of your waking hours. The philosophy about the importance of breakfast probably came from sound logic since it seems an advantage to use awake time to burn off what you consume. First, most of Western society is not nearly as active as prior generations and second, sleep is a 6 to 8 hour fuel burn. Furthermore, when to eat is very much an individual preference based on what the body is communicating. If you feel good and get better body composition results by eating a big breakfast, medium lunch, and light supper, do it. You will also find that time between food consumption becomes less important as a fat burner. I personally know many very lean people, including myself, who seldom eat breakfast, eat a small lunch or snack during the day, and consume most of their food at night. That said, larger nighttime meals should be focused primarily on protein and fat since starches and sugars do need muscle activity to be burned and not be destined for fat deposition. To reiterate, the most important item is the percentage of healthy foods and water intake over the course of a week and manageable nutrition. I formed my eating patterns outlined above due to the evening meal being the easiest to manage because I had time to prepare an outstanding healthy meal, which happens almost every night. It is also a great time to catch up with family or friends. To say this another way, when and how many times you eat must fit into your life and respond to what your body is telling you. Each of us has a little different timing signal from our bodies due to variations in schedule and activity. It makes me pull my hair out when recommendations are given to never skip breakfast, do not eat a lot at night, eat at a certain time, eat 4-6-8 meals a day, or eat 3 squares. These all work, but none have a larger impact than the others when it comes to being lean. It all comes back to what you consume when you choose to consume it.

Portions and Eating Behavior:

In the bustling landscape of Western society, portion sizes often exceed what is necessary, both when dining out and at home. A proactive strategy when eating out to combat this excess is to request a to-go box when placing an order at a restaurant. Place ½ of the meal in it before you eat. This not only assists in managing portion sizes but also affords the luxury of an additional meal from the same dish, promoting both moderation and resourcefulness. Cultivating mindfulness regarding portion sizes is a pivotal component of fostering healthier eating habits, encouraging a shift away from the culture of overindulgence. Portion control becomes much easier when consuming flavorful foods rich in fats, protein, and fiber. The speed at which you consume food affects the final portion eaten. Eating too fast can exceed the speed at which the brain receives feedback and shuts down consumption of food. Most everyone at some point has eaten too much too fast and experienced an uncomfortable distended stomach. The take-home message is to eat great-tasting, nutrient-dense foods at a slower pace. Chewing food is also a very important part of the digestive process. Stop before you are uncomfortable and let the signals in the body tell the brain that you are full and all is well.

Intermittent Fasting:

Embarking on a journey to reconnect with our ancestral eating patterns, intermittent fasting emerges as a beneficial practice. Considering the historical context of humanity's hunting and gathering lifestyle, where longer intervals between meals were the norm, incorporating a weekly 20-hour fasting period can serve as a metabolic reset. For instance, if dinner was consumed at 6 pm the previous night, extending the fasting period until 2 pm the next day can be a manageable and effective practice. This approach taps into the wisdom of our forebearers, contributing not only to metabolic health but also to achieving and maintaining a lean physique.

It's worth noting that the difference between a great meal and an average one can span eight hours, highlighting the significance of the intermittent fasting approach.

Take a Cheat:

The pursuit of leanness doesn't necessitate sacrificing the enjoyment of life's culinary pleasures. Introducing a designated cheat day provides an avenue for indulging in cravings, allowing the consumption of an additional 1000 to 1500 calories of favorite treats. Whether it's savoring the sweetness of donuts, relishing the flavor of beer, or delighting in the comfort of pizza, this day offers a welcome break from the routine, enhancing the overall sustainability of the diet. A cheat day also spikes a hormone called leptin, which has several functions regarding the interaction between hunger and energy balance. To put it simply, a spike in leptin once a week tells your body that all is well and there is plenty of energy. This hormonal message is extremely important in triggering the loss of body fat. Optimal timing for a cheat day involves scheduling it right after an intermittent fast, leveraging metabolic confusion, and mimicking the feast and famine cycles observed in our ancestral heritage. Following this indulgence, returning to the usual dietary management comes with a reset in hormones, contributing to a balanced and sustainable approach to nutrition.

As you embark on your journey through nutrition, always remember the foundation for success...it must be manageable in your life, not manage your life.

Thanks for Reading

Your engagement with this insightful content is greatly appreciated. Consider exploring the website for future subscriptions and upcoming releases, as more valuable content awaits. May these insights guide you on a path of improved health and well-being.

Blessings to You and Yours.

About the Author

In 1972, I was born into a family that had farmed and ranched in Western Nebraska for multiple generations. My brother (Ryan) and my childhood, from the time we were 6 years old until we left home at 18 to go to college, consisted of going to school, working, eating, some extracurricular activities, and sleeping, pretty much in that order.

A lot of the general philosophy of this publication stems from my childhood and other formative experiences in my life. What was evident in my Parents, Grandparents, and Brother, was a good work ethic and prioritizing what is important. Generosity, integrity, and self-sufficiency were at the forefront.

I took on a generalized agricultural major while I figured out what I wanted to do when I grew up. I received my Bachelor's Degree and was given the opportunity to pursue a Master's Degree in animal nutrition. I finished it and was never so glad to see a door close behind me. I disliked school from kindergarten until the completion of my MS, and I still do not know what I want to be when I grow up.

I was an animal nutritionist for about 8 years, working with ranches and feeding operations to help produce meat more efficiently. At this point, I understood a lot about food. After the stint as a nutritionist, at 32, I was given an opportunity to run a company that formulated and produced livestock supplements.

I spent almost 10 years in the production and formulation of livestock feeds. During that time, I led the formulation of somewhere around 5 lines of livestock feeds and am an inventor of a patented supplement for horses. I wanted a change, which is how I have always lived. It happened that one of our partners invested in software that was used to formulate most of the livestock diets in the US that provide meat, milk, and eggs to your table. I ran this company for 10 years until we sold it in 2022.

What now? Reinvent myself. I finally had time to finish this short book and publish it.

I don't care about money or stuff. I care about God, people, and freedom. Unfortunately, freedom does require time, flexibility, and some money. I wrote this publication primarily to help people, but I do appreciate your support of the effort that was put forth to condense a complex subject into a readable book.

www.ingramcontent.com/pod-product-compliance
Lightning Source LLC
Chambersburg PA
CBHW052124030426
42335CB00025B/3099